My Mommom's Market

A Native American Cultural Journey

Coloring Cookbook

by

Dr. June (Charging Spirit) DePonte Sernak

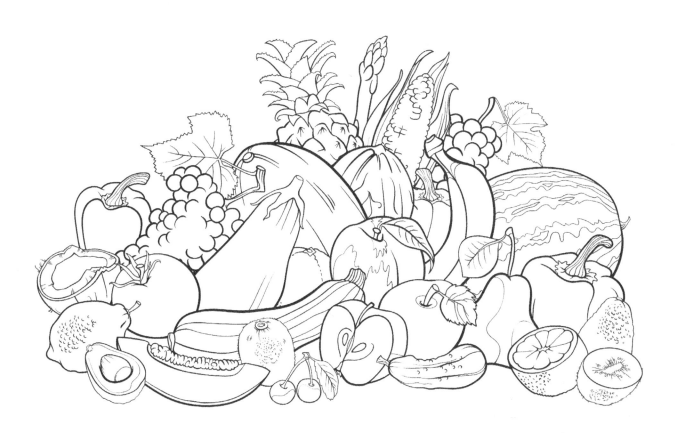

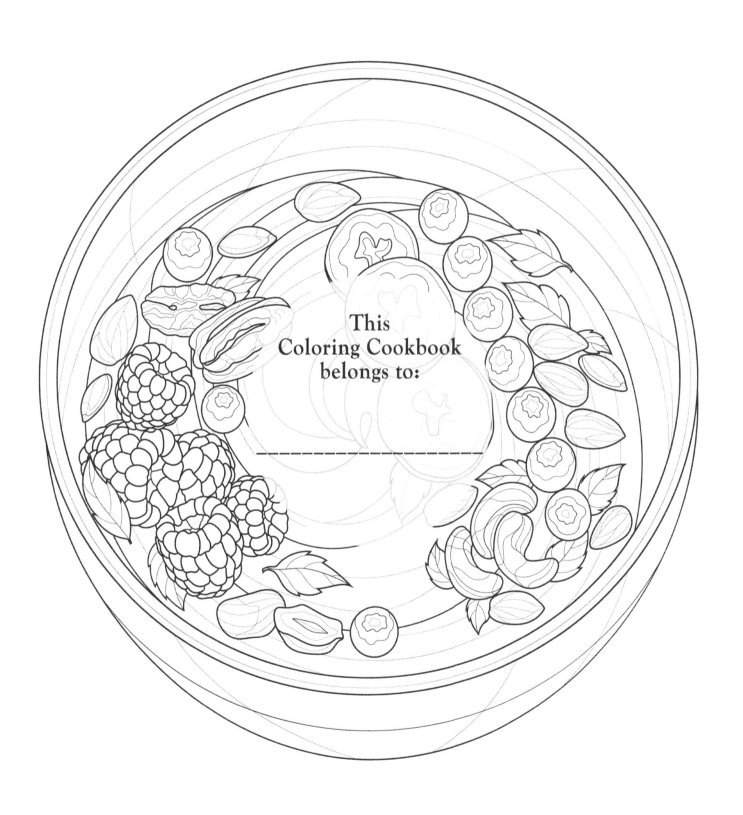

This
Coloring Cookbook
belongs to:

_____

This book is dedicated
to my mommom, my mother, and my daughter.
Thank you for sharing your respect for Mother Earth,
recipes for healing nutrition, and remarkable memories.
Let these recipes feed your family and friends,
heal your heart, and bring joy to your journey.

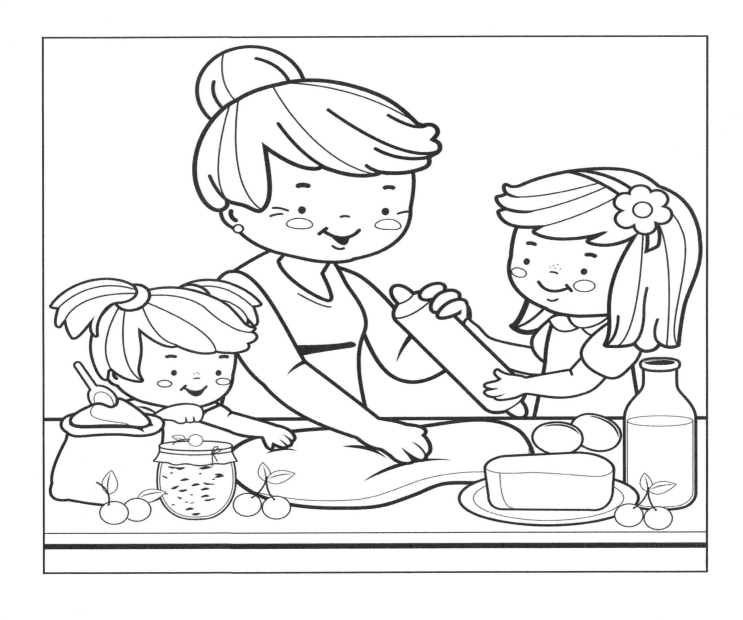

This coloring book was inspired by my grandmother, whom I called Mommom.

My mommom had a market in New Jersey. She sold fresh fruits and vegetables that were grown on the local farms around her. By providing those foods to her customers, my mommom encouraged everyone to take care of each other as they spent time together making and eating delicious food.

Many of the fruits and vegetables my mommom sold were the same our Native American ancestors used in their favorite meals. You can enjoy those same foods today. By doing so, you can honor the Native American cultural heritage and traditions.

Food also provides us with the nutrition we need to be healthy, and cooking with your family or friends is a fun way to connect with them. Then, when eating your meals together, you can tell stories and maybe learn about your ancestors.

I was taught these recipes when I was a little girl. My father brought the fruit and vegetables home from my mommom's market, and my mother would cook each recipe. I learned from her, and now it's your turn to learn.

Make this cookbook your own. Color it in ways that make your heart smile. Learn to make each recipe with an adult and share it with your family and friends. Then have more fun finding new ways to eat healthy fruits and vegetables.

I hope you enjoy making these as much as I did.

Wishing you love and health,

Dr. June

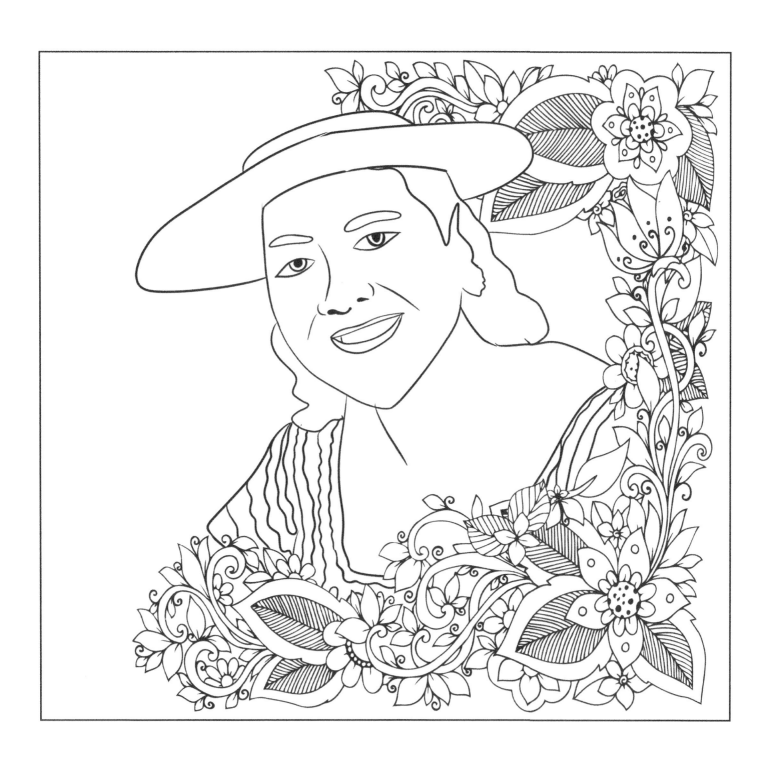

Recipe Index

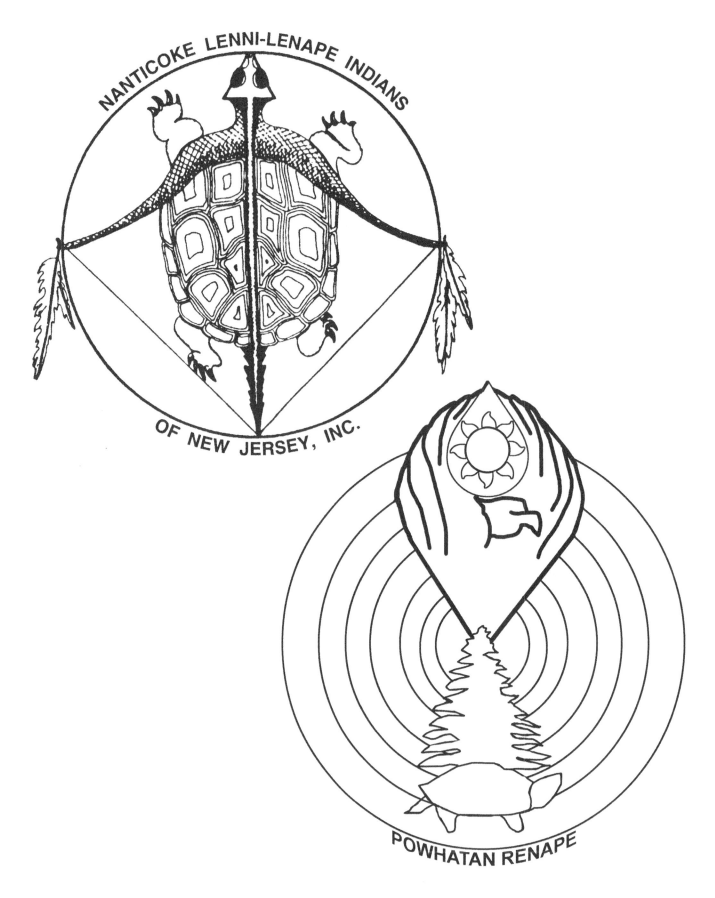

My Native American ancestors came from the Nanticoke Lenni-Lenape and Powhatan Renape nations.

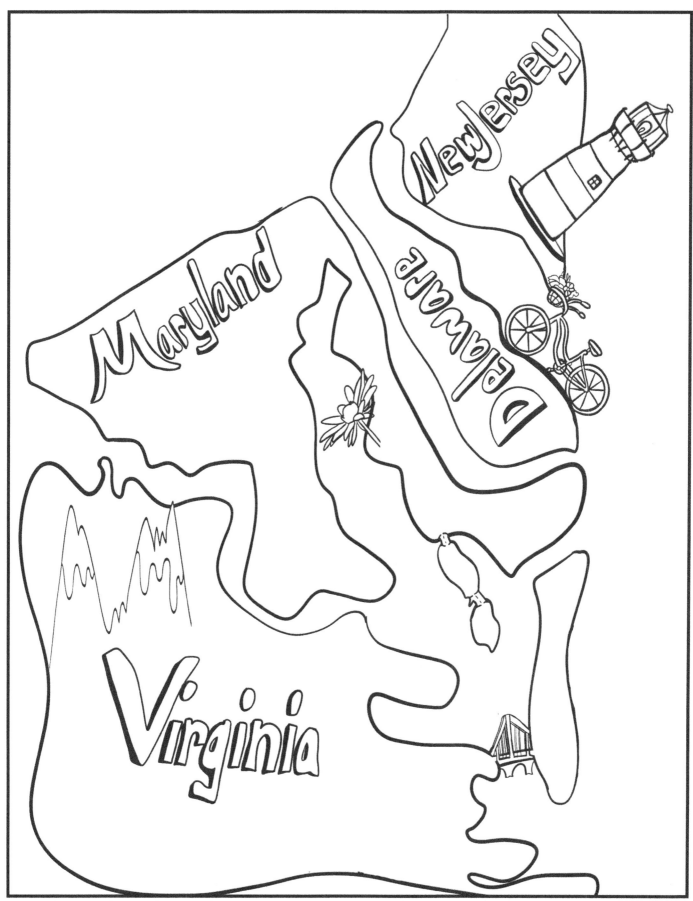

Nehemiah and Sarah Carney, my great-great grandparents, moved from Virginia to Delaware to New Jersey

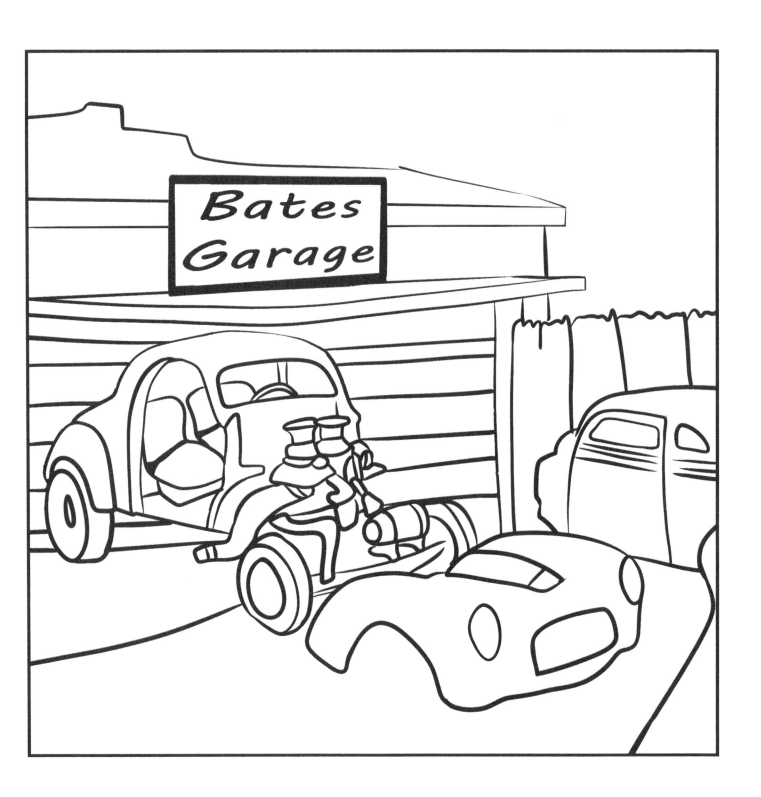

My grandparents were Gladys and William. They moved to Haddonfield,
New Jersey, where my grandfather fixed cars in his shop called
"Bates Garage."

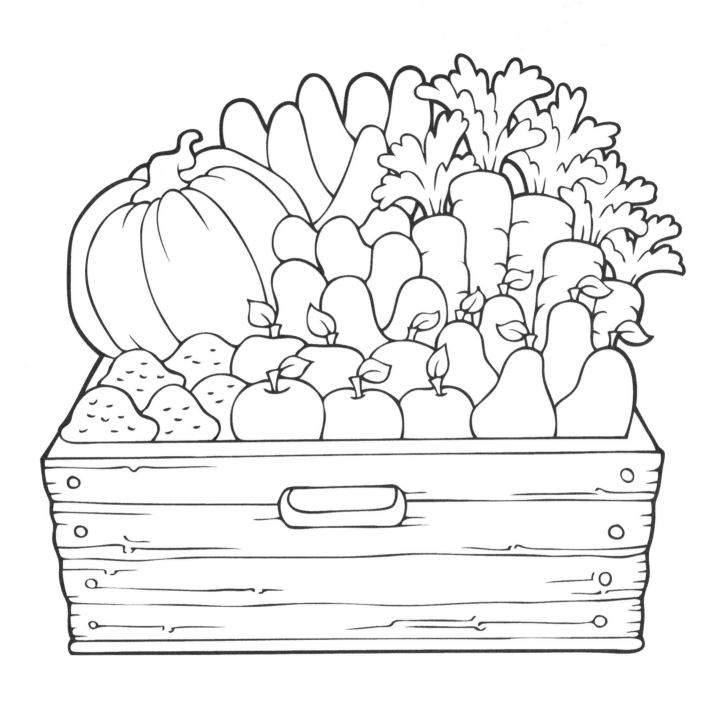

His shop later became the perfect place for Mommom to set up her market. She sold corn, tomatoes, asparagus, berries, and many other Jersey crops.

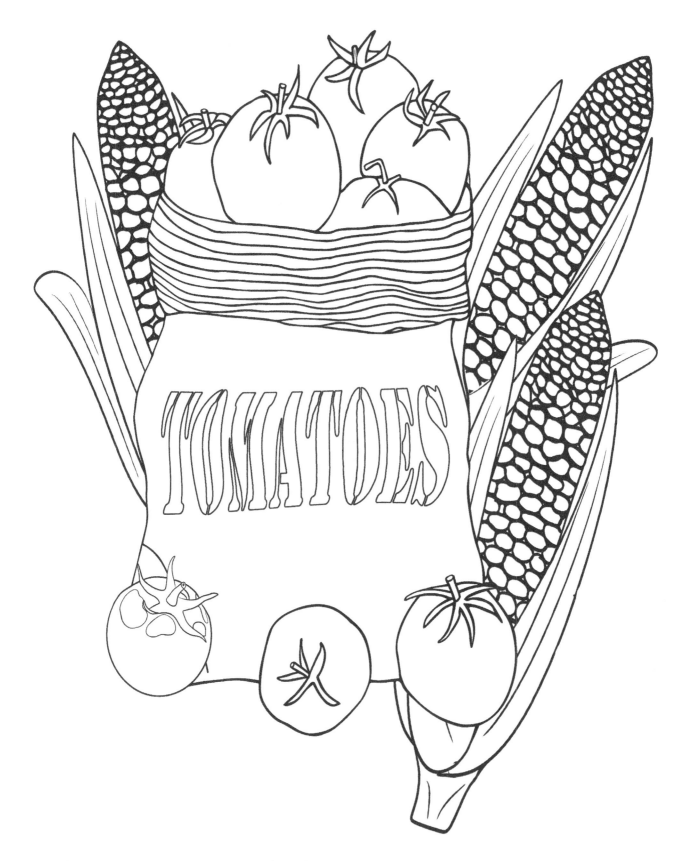

In the summer, she would sell as many as 2,000 ears of corn and 450 pounds of tomatoes! My grandfather drove to many farms in South Jersey to bring the fruits and vegetables to her market.

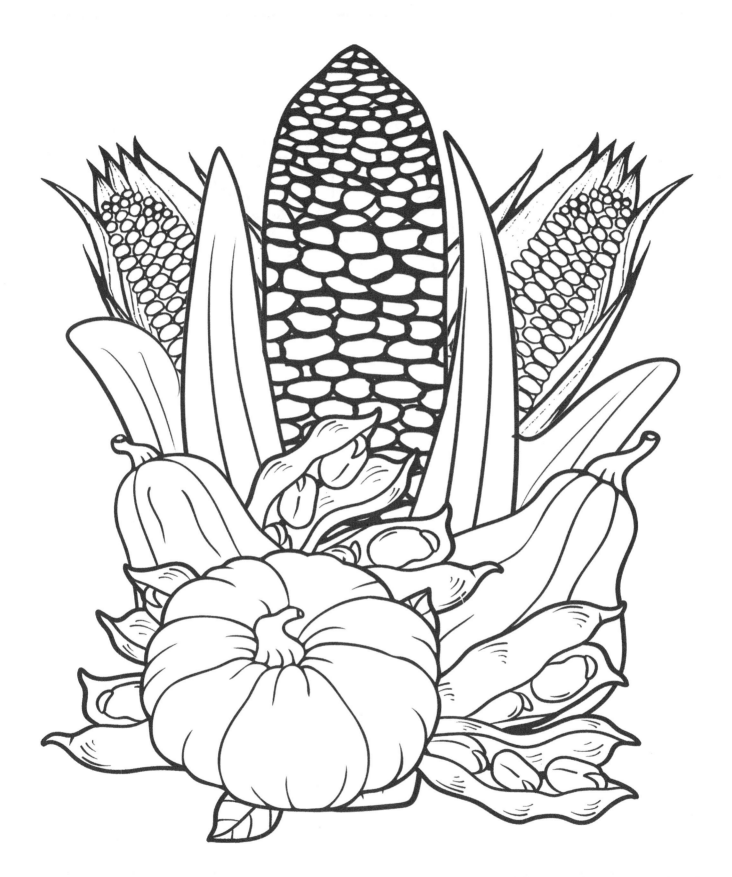

Mommom was most proud to sell corn, squash, and beans because that's what clan mothers from ancient times have always fed their families. They are full of nutrients that kept our ancestors healthy and keep us healthy.

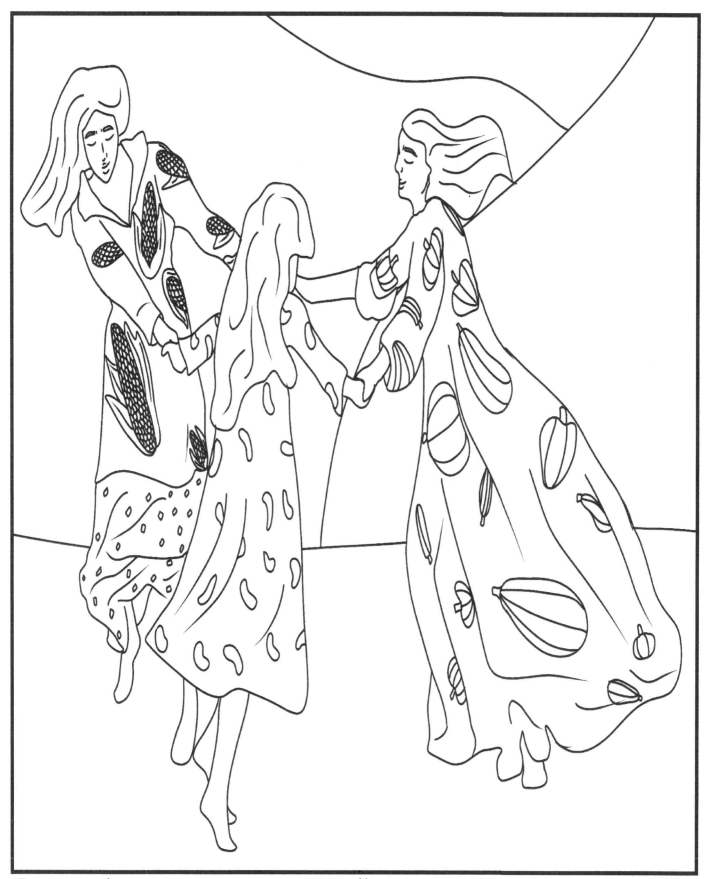

Because they are so important, we call corn, squash, and beans the Three Sisters. We eat them in many different ways and always have them on the table for our holidays.

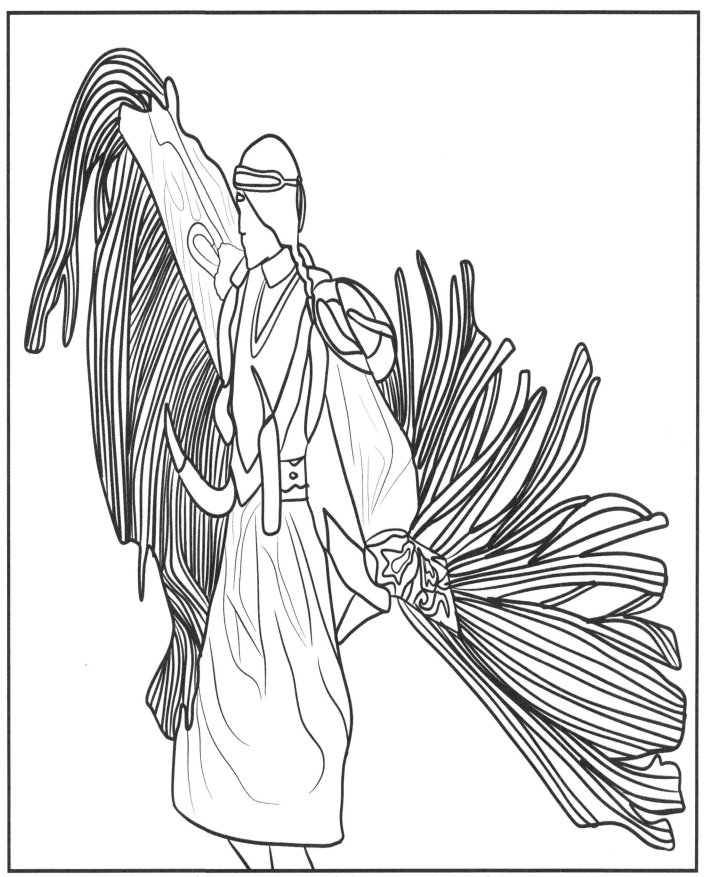

Each gathering and holiday, we celebrate with food from Mother Earth. We pay our respect to the harvest through rituals such as Powwows and prayers, the same way our ancestors did.

Succotash

Succotash is a vegetable dish combining corn and lima beans together. There are two recipes listed here. One is the traditional way of making succotash, which calls for fresh vegetables and salt pork. When it's hard to find fresh ingredients, or you need a quicker process, use the recipe for modern succotash.

This recipe honors my cousin and Nanticoke Lenni-Lenape Tribal member, Gail (Gentle Leaves) Gould. Her love not only enhanced her succotash but provided nourishment and comfort to all who loved her.

Traditional Succotash

Ingredients:
- 1 ½ pounds salt pork
- 1 dozen ears of corn
- 1 basket of lima beans
- alt, pepper, sugar to taste (approximately ¼ to ½ tsp each)

Directions:
- Boil salt pork for 30 minutes.
- Shell beans (remove from the hard outer shell) Place in a colander and wash thoroughly.
- Place beans and seasonings in a large saucepan, add water, covering the beans by two to three inches.
- Bring to a boil, then reduce heat and simmer for 60 minutes or until tender.
- While beans cook, shuck and clean corn, then cut corn from the cobb.
- Stand corn upright on a cutting board. Cut corn off of the cobb with a small sharp knife from top of ear moving downward.
- Add kernels of corn to beans and continue to cook for another 10-15 minutes.
- Season to taste (1/4 teaspoon of salt for desired taste) and enjoy.

* Corn on the cob grows in a shell called a husk. We call the process of peeling the husk, shucking. Once the husk is peeled, it can be thrown away, and the ears of corn can be cleaned of any remaining threads).

Modern Succotash:

Ingredients:

- 6 slices of bacon
- 12-ounce bag of frozen or 15.25-ounce can of lima beans
- 12-ounce whole kernel or 15.25-ounce can whole-kernel corn
- 2 Tbs butter
- ¼ tsp of salt, ¼ tsp of garlic powder for seasoning

Directions:

- Fry the bacon in a pan until done. Remove slices and set aside to drain on paper towels and reserve the grease.
- Defrost the beans and corn if using frozen, then drain until dry. (If canned, drain fully, then pat dry with a clean paper towel.)
- Add the beans and corn to the reserved bacon grease.
- Add the bacon back to the beans and corn mixture and season with ¼ teaspoon of salt and garlic powder to taste.
- Heat on low for 15 minutes, stirring gently.
- Add 2 Tbs of butter to the mixture until fully melted. Stir thoroughly, then enjoy.

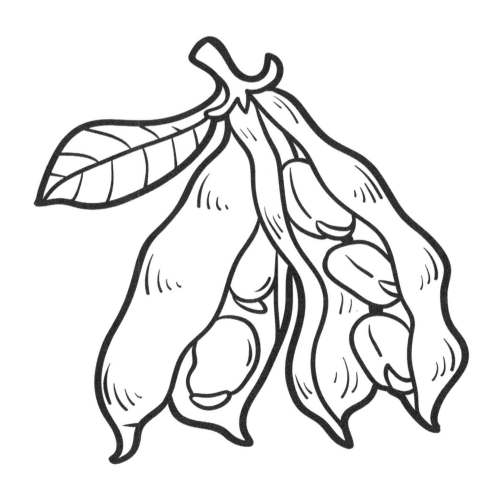

Zucchini Squash Bread

Ingredients:

- 3 cups flour
- 1 ½ cups sugar
- 1 ½ tsp. cinnamon
- 1 tsp salt
- 1 tsp baking powder
- ¾ tsp baking soda
- 1 cup raisins*
- 1 cup chopped nuts*
- 2 cups shredded zucchini squash
- 3 eggs
- 1 cup of oil
- 1 tsp. vanilla

Directions:

- Preheat oven to 350 degrees.
- In a large bowl, stir together all dry ingredients and squash.
- In a separate bowl, beat eggs, then add in the oil and vanilla.
- Pour the mixed wet ingredients over the flour mixture and stir until mixed well.
- Bake in a greased loaf pan for 1 ½ hours at 350 degrees.
- Cool in pan for 10 minutes and invert on wax paper to serve.

*Raisins and chopped nuts are optional to preference

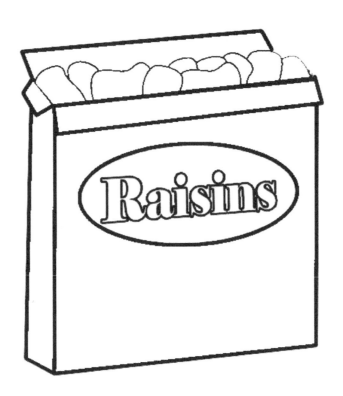

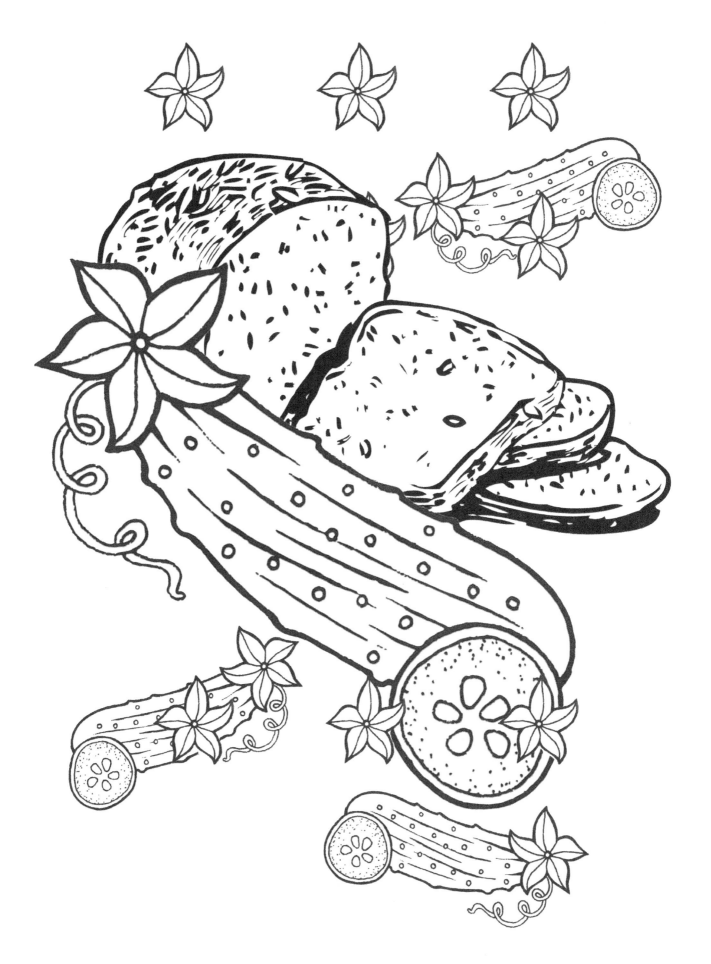

13

Corn Pudding

Ingredients:

- 3 eggs, well beaten
- 2 cups corn kernels*
- ¼ cup flour
- ½ tsp pepper
- 1 tbl sugar
- 1/3 cup of butter, melted
- 1 tsp salt
- 2 cups light cream

Directions:

- Preheat the oven to 325 degrees.
- Mix the dry ingredients and add corn.
- Combine the melted butter with the light cream, and add to the corn mixture, mixing together thoroughly.
- Pour all into a 1 ½ quart baking dish set inside a larger baking pan. Pour about 1 inch of water into the larger pan.
- Set large pan with water and baking dish in the preheated oven.
- Bake for 60 minutes or until the top feels firm and is browned.

*Corn kernels can be canned or frozen. Drain and dry before adding to dry ingredients.

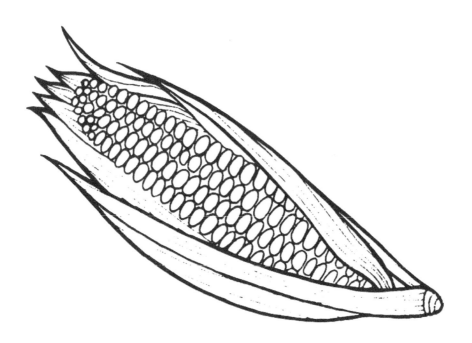

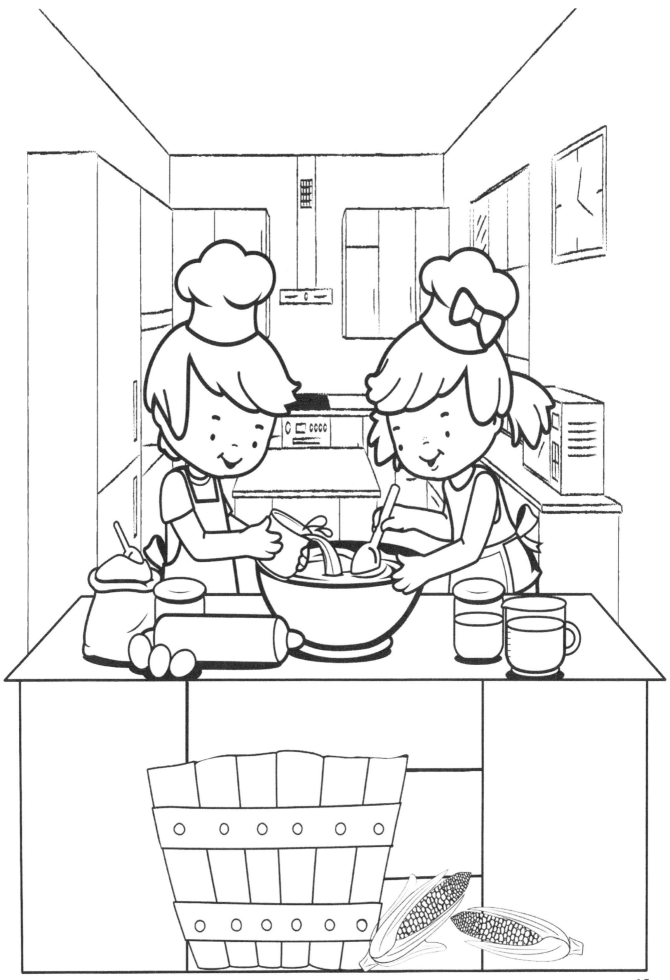

15

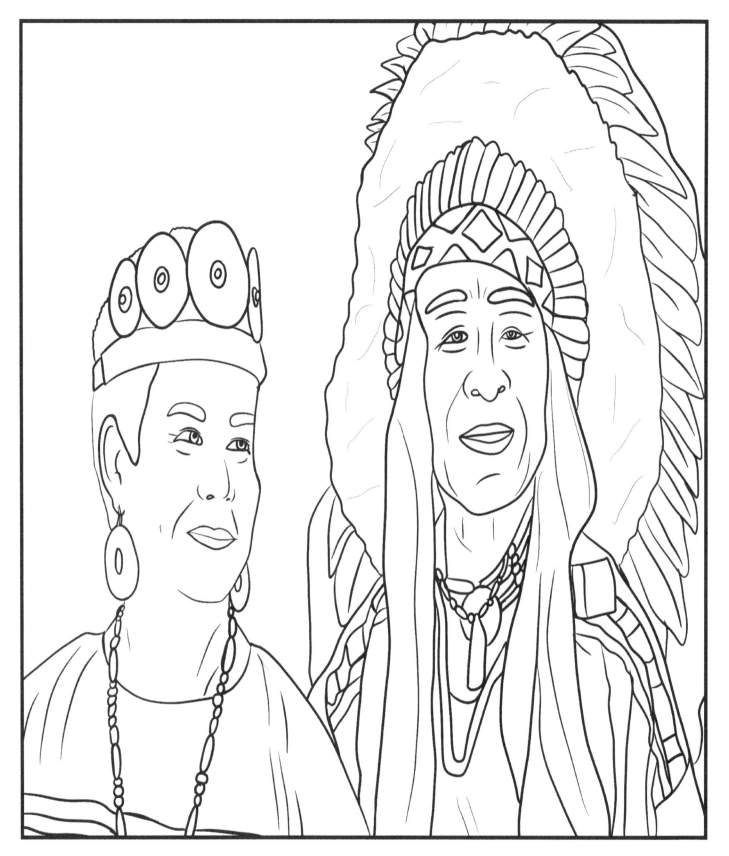

We honor our elders for the wisdom they pass down to us. Our family traditions and favorite recipes come from our ancestors.
They teach us to appreciate everything that comes from Mother Earth and not to waste food.

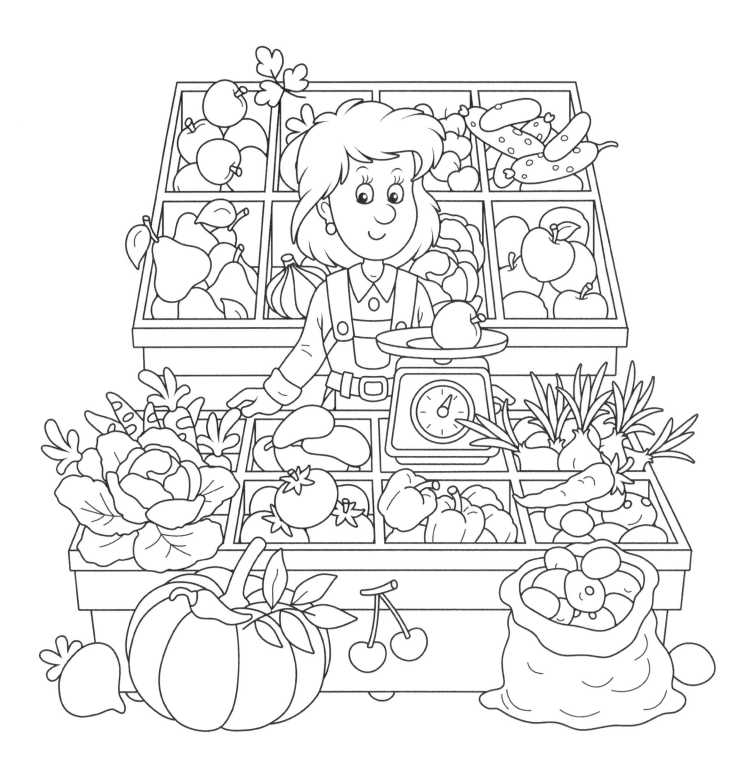

Clan Mothers, like my mommom, are respected and honored for their wisdom. Not only do they gather and prepare food to keep us healthy, but they also choose the tribal chiefs and make many important decisions in our nations.

Traditional Fried Chicken

Ingredients:

- 2 pounds chicken (individual packages of chicken breast, thighs, and drums sticks with skin work best and are easier than carving a full chicken)
- Flour
- Salt and Pepper
- Lard, bacon drippings, or vegetable oil

Directions:

- Rinse and cut the chicken into serving pieces, drain, and pat dry with a paper towel.
- Fill a large frying pan with about 2 inches of lard (oil)—enough to cover the chicken.
- Sprinkle salt and pepper over the chicken and dredge it in flour to cover all sides well (alternatively, you can place chicken, flour, and seasonings in a Ziploc bag, seal to close, and shake until covered).
- When lard (oil) is hot, place chicken in a pan with skin side down.
- Cook until chicken is brown on one side, then turn to brown the other side.
- Once browned, lower the heat and continue to cook until done.*

*Note: chicken is not safe to eat until the internal temperature is 165 degrees.

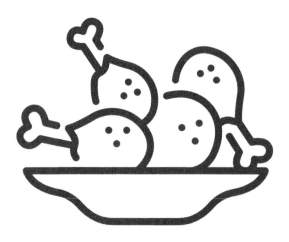

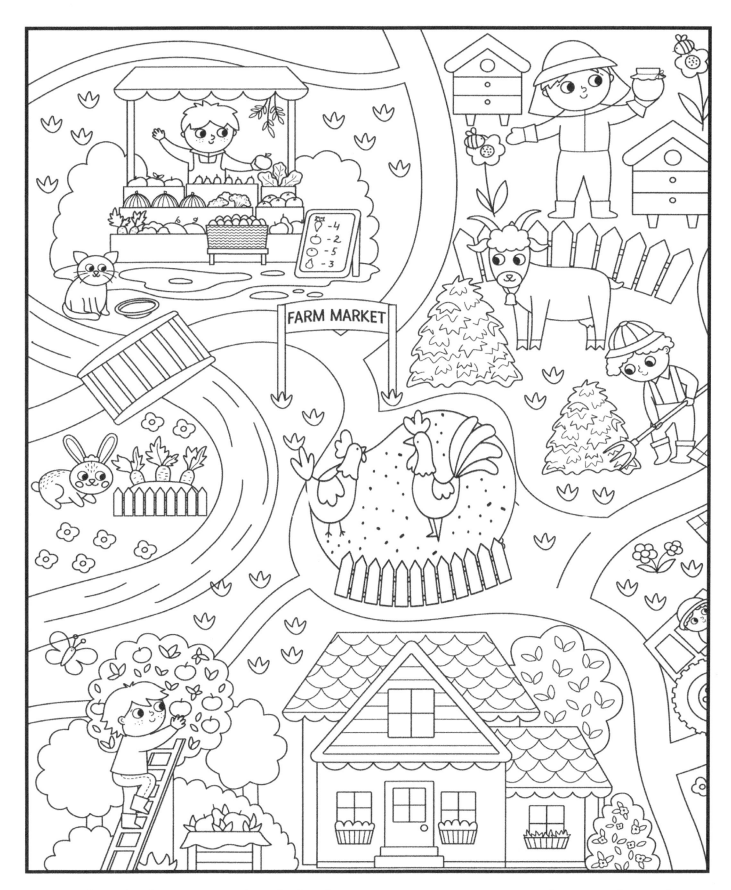

One family favorite is fried chicken. My mommom taught me about how chickens were raised on farms. The lard she used to cook our chicken came from the pork fat she saved and collected in a jar placed on the sink.

Potato Salad

Ingredients:

- 10 medium white potatoes
- 1 small onion
- 4 celery sticks
- 2-3 hard-boiled eggs
- 1 Tbs celery seed
- salt & pepper
- ½ cup mayonnaise
- 2 Tbs mustard
- 1 Tbs celery seed
- a pinch of sugar
- ¼ tsp of paprika and ¼ tsp of dried parsley (for garnish on top before serving)

Directions:

- Peel and dice potatoes and place in pot.
- Cover with water and place pot on stove. Bring water to a boil; cook potatoes in boiling water until they are tender. Use a fork to test potatoes by gently spearing them. The fork should cut through easily.
- Drain the liquid and place the potatoes in a bowl. Let them cool.
- Dice celery and onion and chop eggs.
- Gently mix all ingredients (except garnishes), being careful not to mash the potatoes.
- Sprinkle garnishes on top.

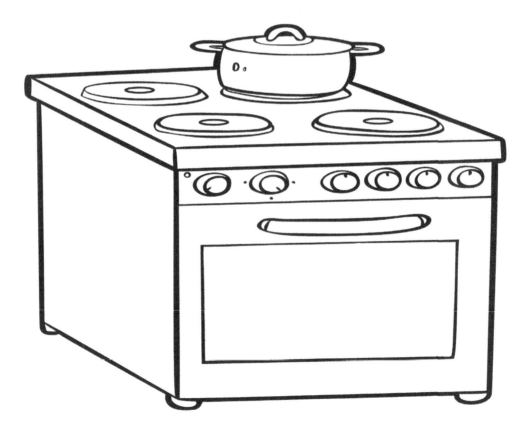

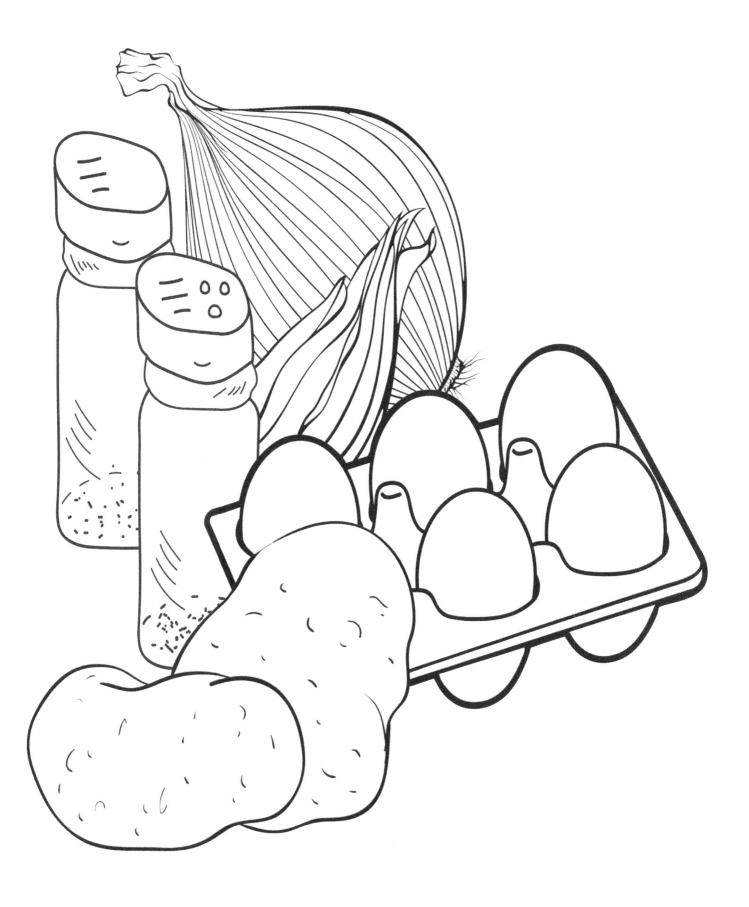

Another family favorite is potato salad. It goes well with fried chicken and corn on the cob.

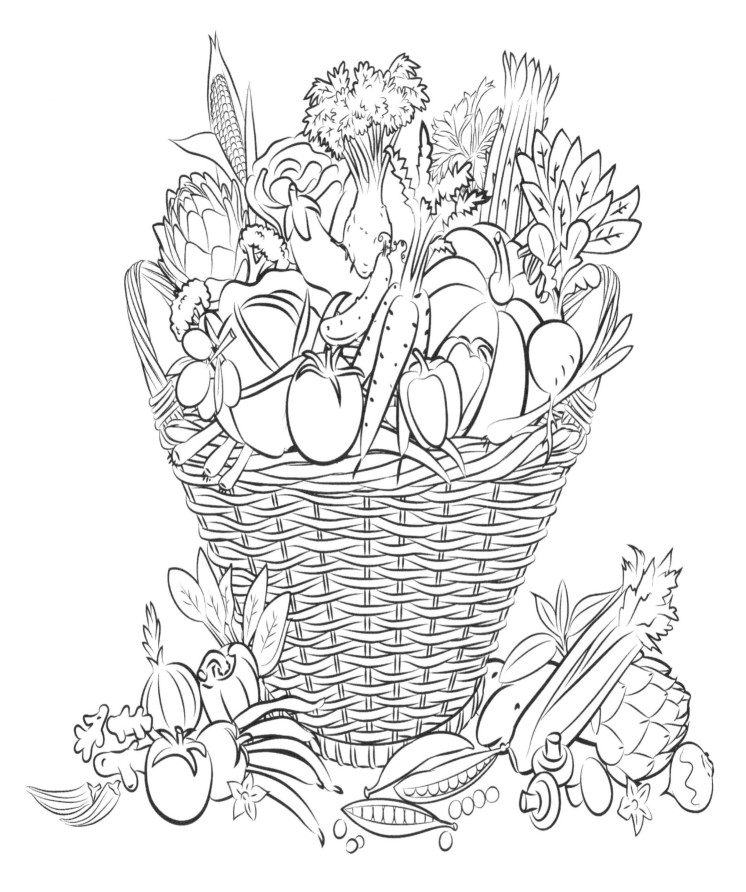

My mommom worked in her market with my grandfather.
They were married for over sixty years. The market was always full of the
vibrant colors of the seasonal harvests.

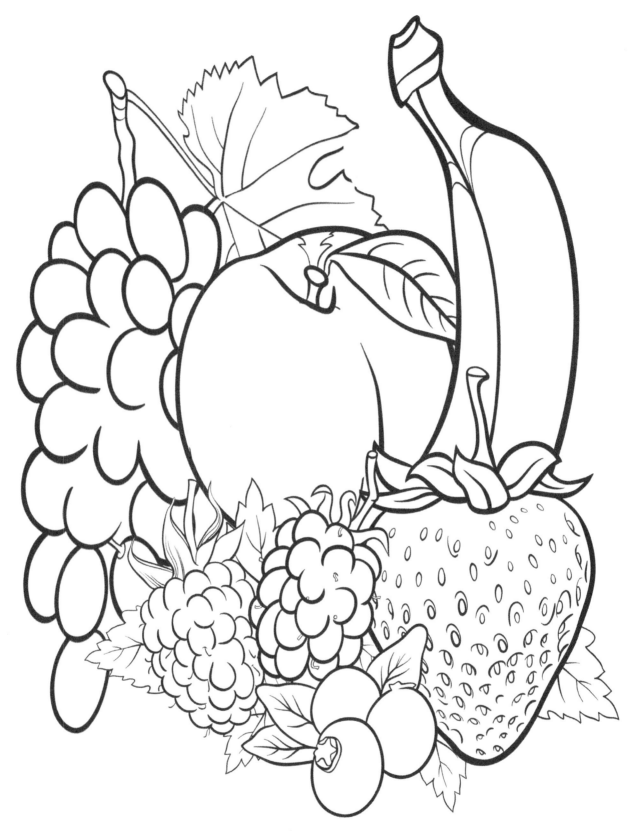

My favorite season was summer when the fruit came. In May, there were
strawberries. In June, we had blueberries. Then in July, we received peaches.
After dinner, we liked to have a little something sweet,
so we made delicious desserts with these fruits!

Strawberry Shortcake

Biscuits

Ingredients:

- 2 cups of flour
- 1 tsp of salt
- 1 Tbs of shortening
- 1 Tbs of baking powder
- 1 Tbs of sugar
- 6 Tbs of unsalted butter
- ¾ cup of milk (whole or 2%)

Directions:

- Preheat oven to 350 degrees.
- Grease and flour a baking sheet.
- Mix the dry ingredients together.
- Cut butter into small pieces and add to the dry mixture, stirring in until the mixture becomes course crumbles.
- Add milk and stir until thoroughly combined.
- Section pieces of dough (palm size) and roll until round.
- Bake for 20 minutes.
- (Biscuits can also be made from store options such as Pillsbury Grands. Follow instructions on the package and continue the recipe.)

Strawberries

Ingredients:

- 2 pints of strawberries
- ¼ teaspoon of sugar

Directions:

- Clean strawberries, drain, and cut in quarters.
- Place in a bowl. Add sugar and stir gently.
- Cut a warm biscuit in half, longways.
- Spoon a layer of strawberries onto the bottom of the biscuit.
- Cover with the top of the biscuit.
- Place another layer of strawberries on top.
- Serve warm with vanilla ice cream or whipped cream for a special extra treat.

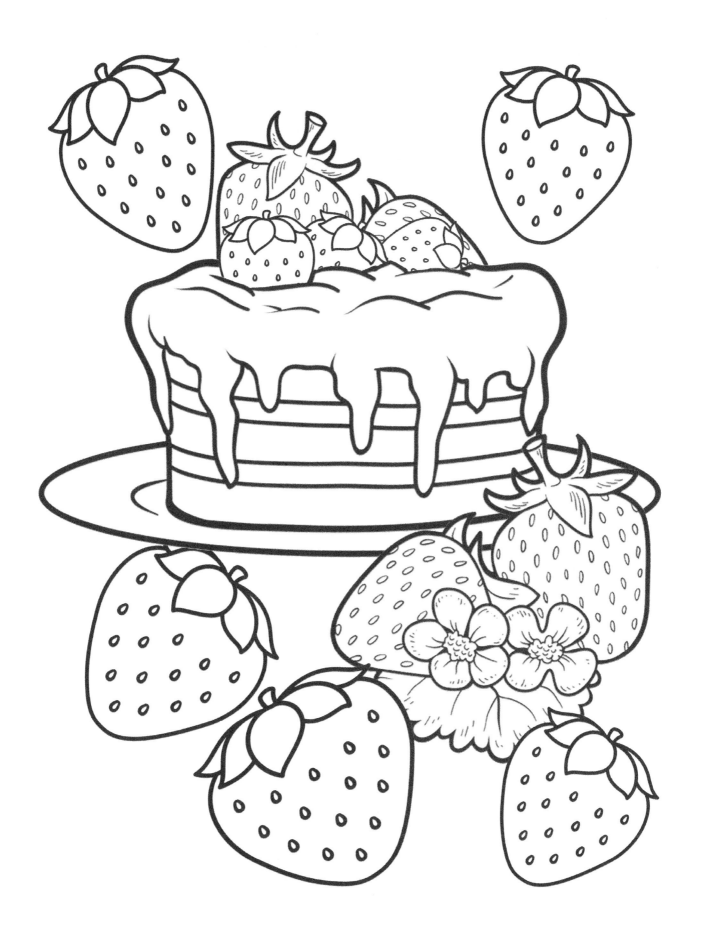

Blueberry Buckle

Ingredients:

- 2 cups all-purpose flour
- 2 tsp baking powder
- ½ tsp salt
- ¼ cup unsalted butter
- ¾ cup white sugar
- 1 large egg
- ½ cup milk
- 2 ½ cups fresh blueberries
- ½ cup white sugar
- ⅓ cup all-purpose flour
- ½ tsp ground cinnamon
- ¼ cup unsalted butter, softened

Directions:

- Preheat oven to 350 degrees.
- Grease and flour a springform pan.
- Sift 2 cups flour, baking powder, and salt into a bowl.
- Beat ¼ cup butter, ¾ cup sugar, and egg with an electric mixer in a large bowl until smooth.
- Gradually add milk and beat until fluffy; stir in flour mixture, making a stiff batter.
- Gently fold in blueberries and spread batter into prepared springform pan.
- Mix ½ cup sugar, 1/3 cup flour, cinnamon, and ¼ cup butter in a bowl until blended and crumbly in texture. Sprinkle on top of batter, then lightly press topping into batter using fingertips.
- Bake in preheated oven until golden and a toothpick inserted in the middle comes out with moist crumbs, about 40 minutes.

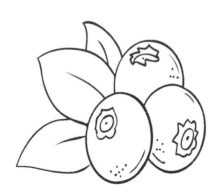

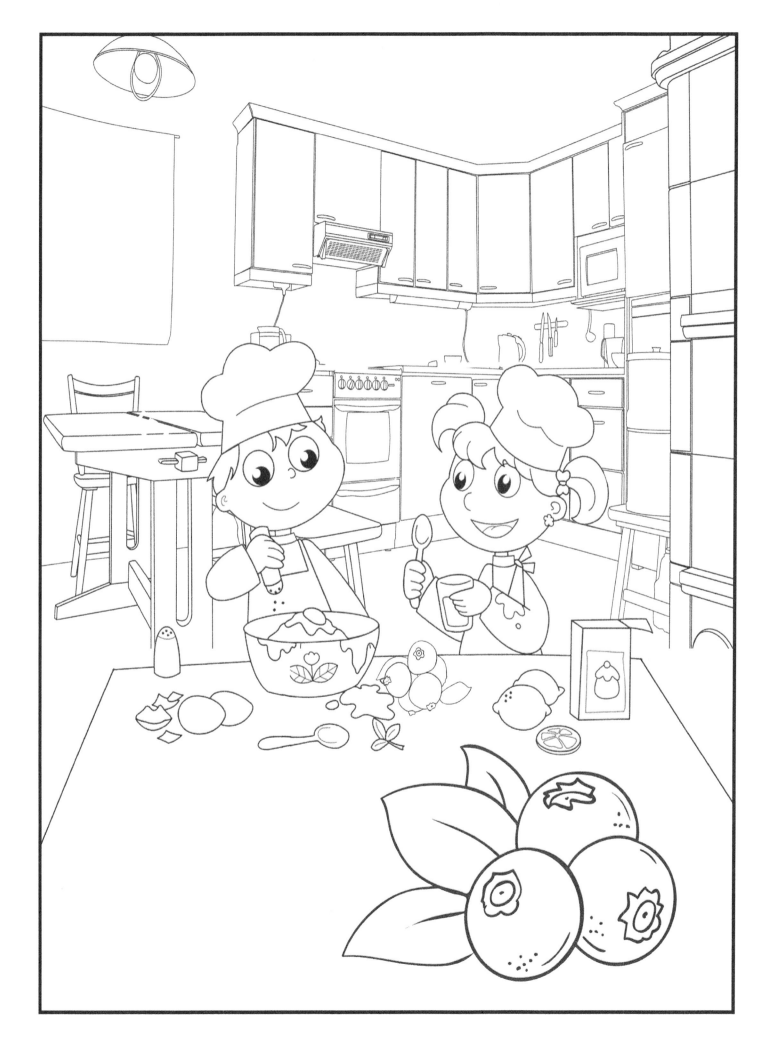

Peach Cobbler

Ingredients:

- 1 cup original Bisquick® mix
- 1 cup milk
- ½ teaspoon ground nutmeg
- ½ cup butter or margarine, melted
- 1 cup sugar
- 6 sliced peaches

Directions:

- Preheat the oven to 350 degrees.
- Stir together Bisquick mix, milk, and nutmeg in an ungreased 8x8-inch baking dish.
- Stir in melted butter or margarine until blended.
- Stir together peaches and sugar in a bowl until combined; spoon over batter.
- Bake in the preheated oven until golden, 50 to 60 minutes.

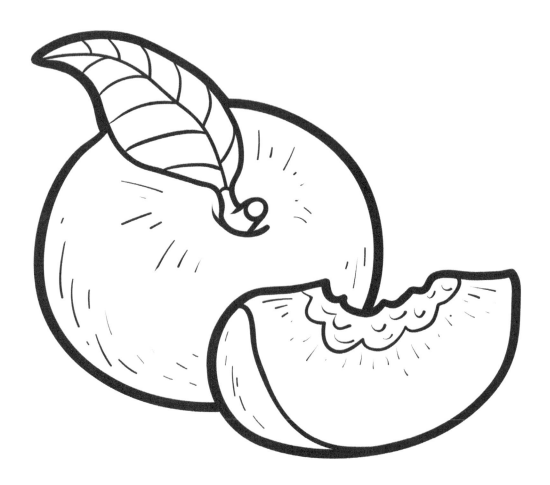

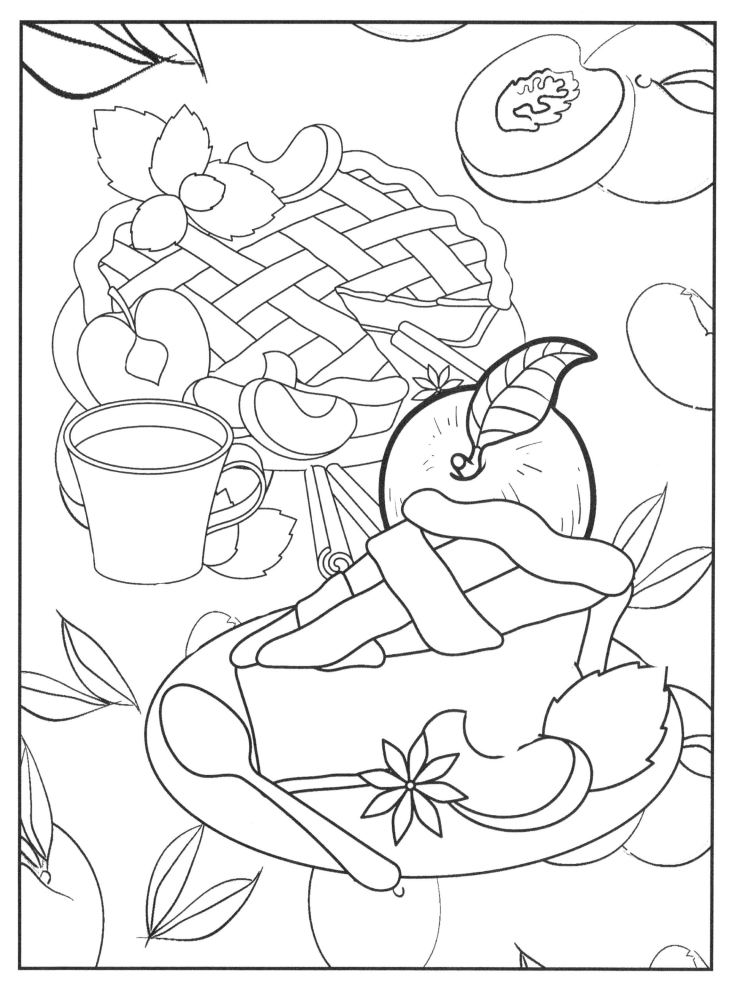

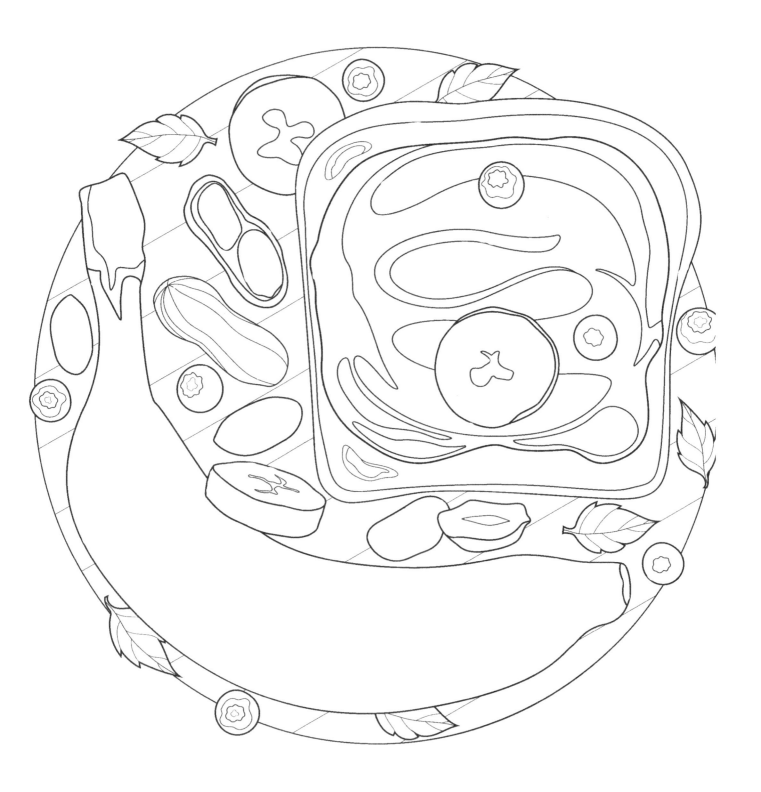

Fresh fruit and vegetables also make wonderful treats and snacks.
Strawberries, bananas, blueberries, peaches, and apples go well with
peanut butter.

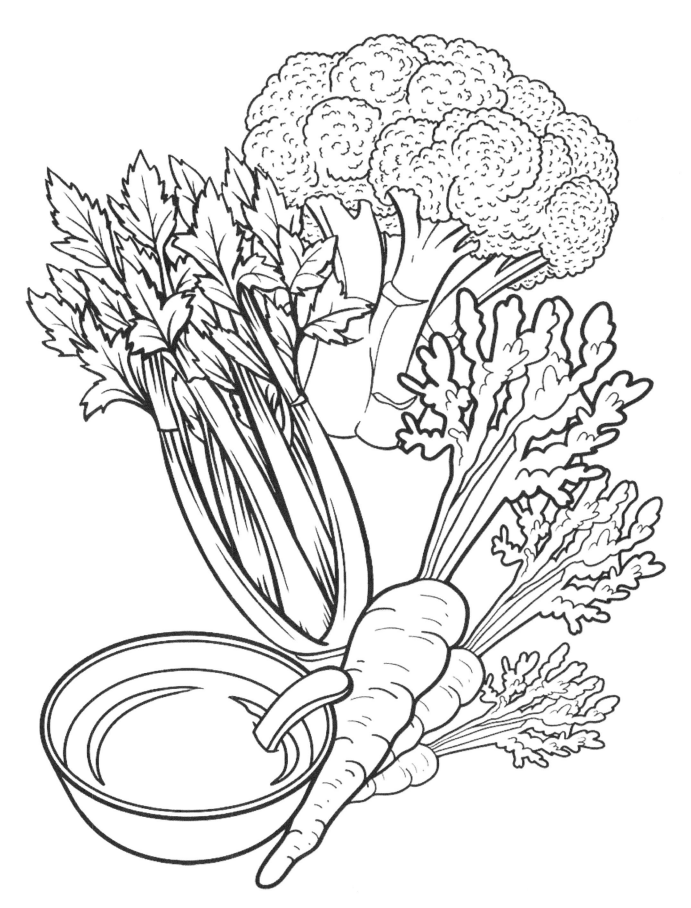

Raw carrots, broccoli, and celery are healthy and delicious snacks and go
well with cream cheese or low-fat ranch dressing.

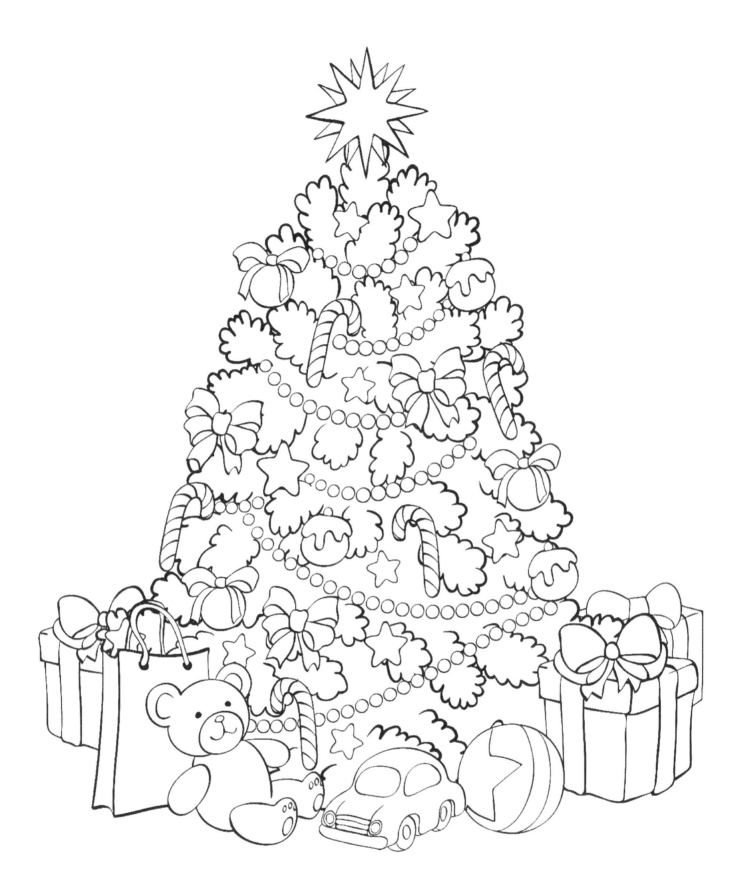

In the fall and winter, Mommom sold wreaths and Christmas trees in her market. Christmas was my mommom's favorite holiday. She would get the biggest tree she could find for her home and place it by the front window.

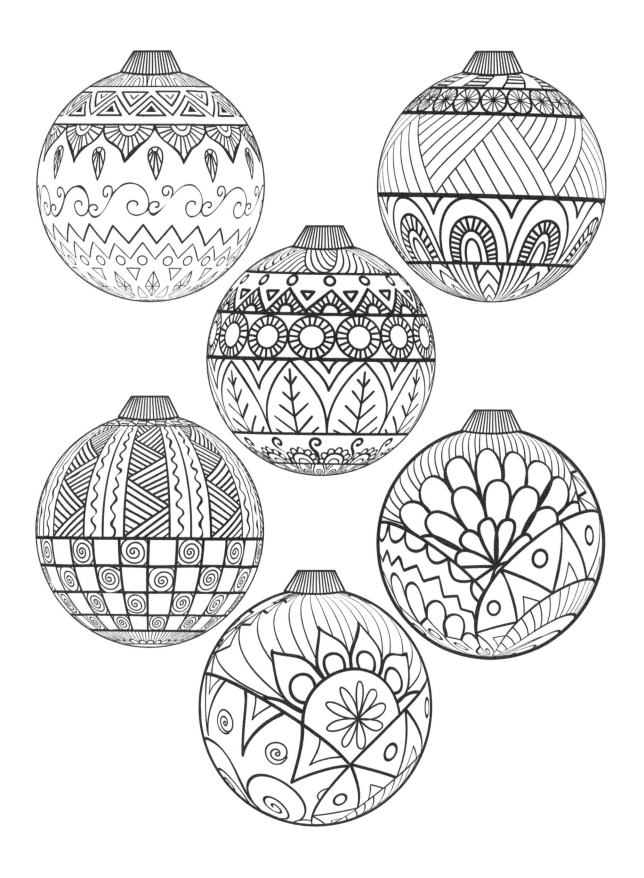

Mommom's favorite color was pink. She would decorate her tree with large pink ornaments.

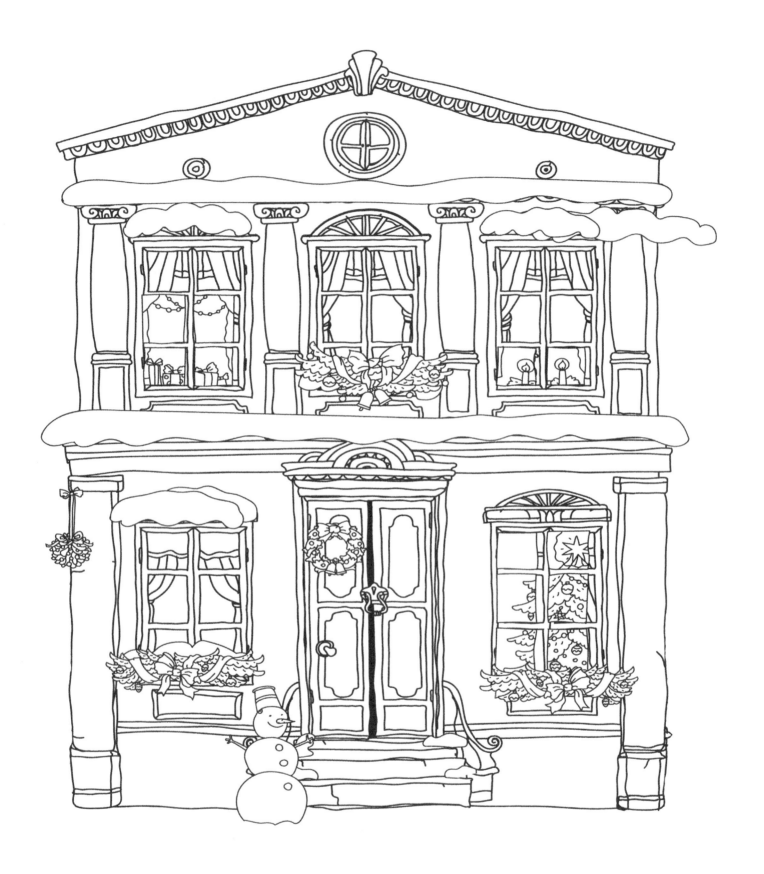

My favorite part of Christmas was when my grandparents would drive
my cousins and me around at night to look at all the decorated
houses and holiday lights.

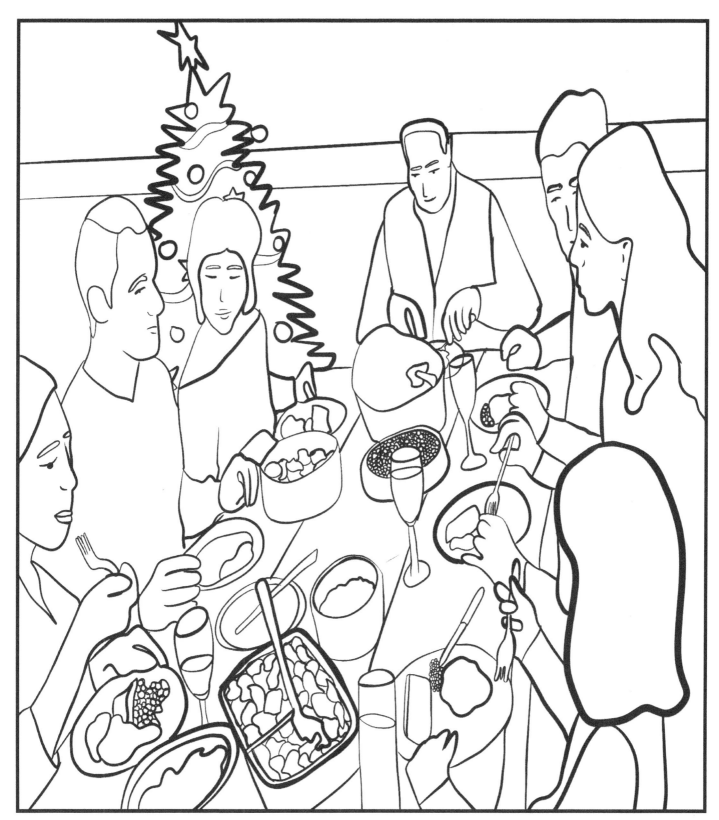

I also loved when my aunts, uncles, and cousins would join my family at my grandparents for a big Christmas meal. We would laugh and share stories about our heritage and culture. Afterward, we played music and enjoyed holiday songs. My grandmother enjoyed singing in her church choir and would share her musical talents with our family.

Pineapple Stuffing

Ingredients

- ½ cup whipped butter or softened margarine
- 1 cup white sugar
- 4 eggs
- 1 (20-ounce) can crushed pineapple, drained
- 5 slices white bread, cubed

Directions

- Preheat the oven to 350 degrees.
- Grease a 9-inch baking pan.
- Cream margarine and sugar together in a mixing bowl with an electric hand mixer.
- Beat in eggs one at a time until blended thoroughly.
- With a large spoon, stir in the pineapple to mix.
- Place bread cubes in the baking dish. Place the mixture over the bread cubes in the baking dish.
- Bake in the preheated oven for 1 hour or until brown. Let it sit a few minutes to firm up before serving.

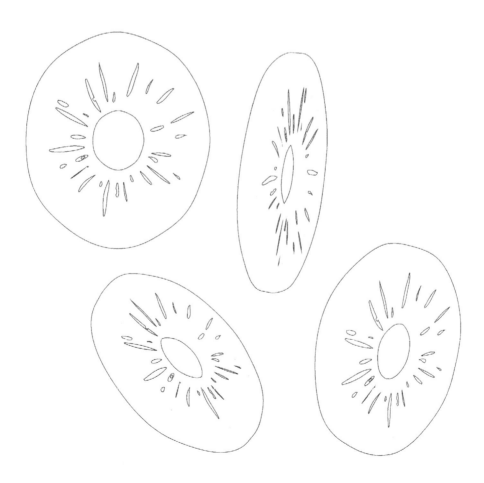

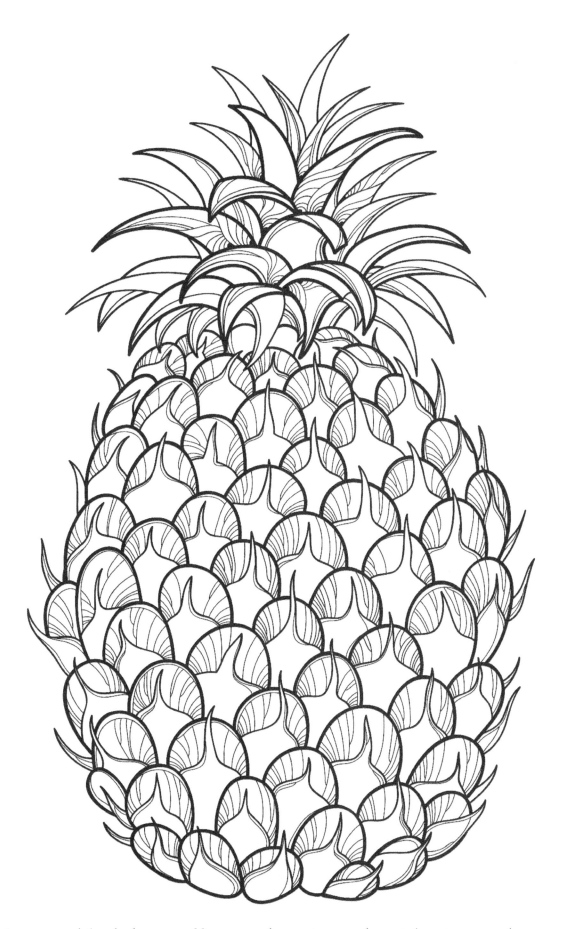

A special holiday stuffing we love is made with pineapples.

Candied Yams

Ingredients:

- 2 ½ pounds yams
- 2 tablespoons butter
- 2 cups brown sugar
- 1 cup orange juice
- 1 teaspoon ground nutmeg
- 3 cups marshmallows

Directions:

- Preheat the oven to 400 degrees.
- Roast whole yams for 35 to 40 minutes or until heated through and soft. Test with a fork to spear yams to check if they are tender.
- Reduce the oven heat to 350 degrees.
- Melt butter in a large pot over medium heat. Stir brown sugar, orange juice, and nutmeg into the melted butter to dissolve the sugar completely; bring to a boil, reduce heat to low, and cook until the liquid thickens into a syrup, about 10 to 15 minutes.
- Peel cooled yams and cut into bite-sized chunks; arrange in a single layer in a 13x9-inch baking dish.
- Drizzle syrup over the yams.
- Bake in the preheated oven, twice opening the oven to spoon syrup over the yams, until the chunks are fork-tender, about 35 minutes.
- Spread marshmallows over the yams and continue baking until the marshmallows are puffy and browned, about 10 minutes more.

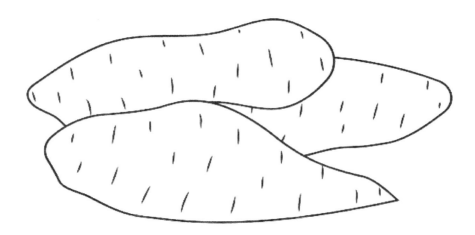

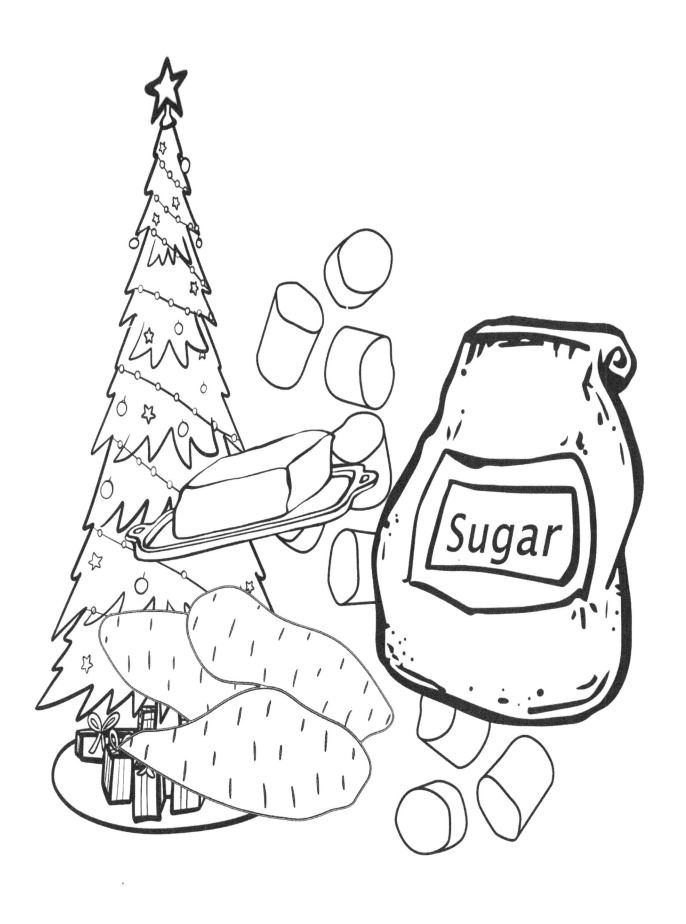

One of my favorite holiday treats is candied yams.

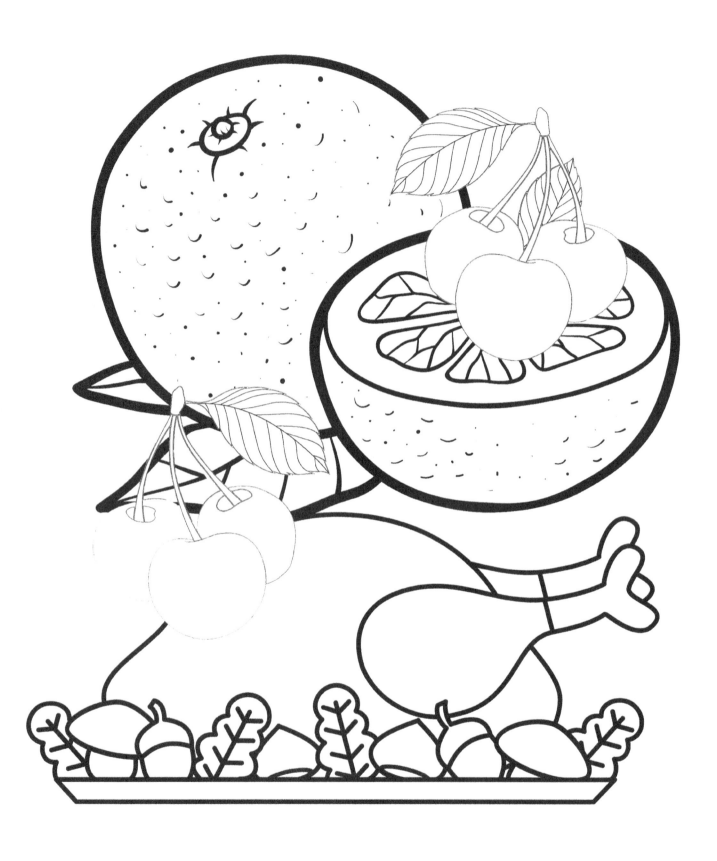

At Thanksgiving and Christmas, we would make orange baskets. Cut the top of the orange into a basket handle shape and add cherries.

The Powhatan Renape Nation came to southern New Jersey in the late 1800s. We remain a strong community, sharing stories about the difficulties of our ancestors as we celebrate their traditions and spiritual values. Through sharing our stories and recipes with each new generation, we continue to keep our legacy alive.

New Jersey is home to two other Native American Tribes, including the Ramapough Tribe in northern New Jersey and the Nanticoke Lenni-Lenape Tribe in southern New Jersey. We share our culture through events such as Powwows, where we include spiritual dances and prayer services passed down to us from our ancestors. We also share in food made from recipes used over many years by tribes around the country.

Other Native Americans around the country follow similar rituals as the Powhatan Renape Nation, such as wearing traditional clothing like jingle dresses. Jingle dresses are used in dance ceremonies during Powwows to pray for family members and ancestors. The dances are also ways to pay respect to Mother Earth and appreciation for the harvest that provides the food we eat.

Similarly, through this coloring book, my mommom's market lives on in our meals, holidays, and prayers.

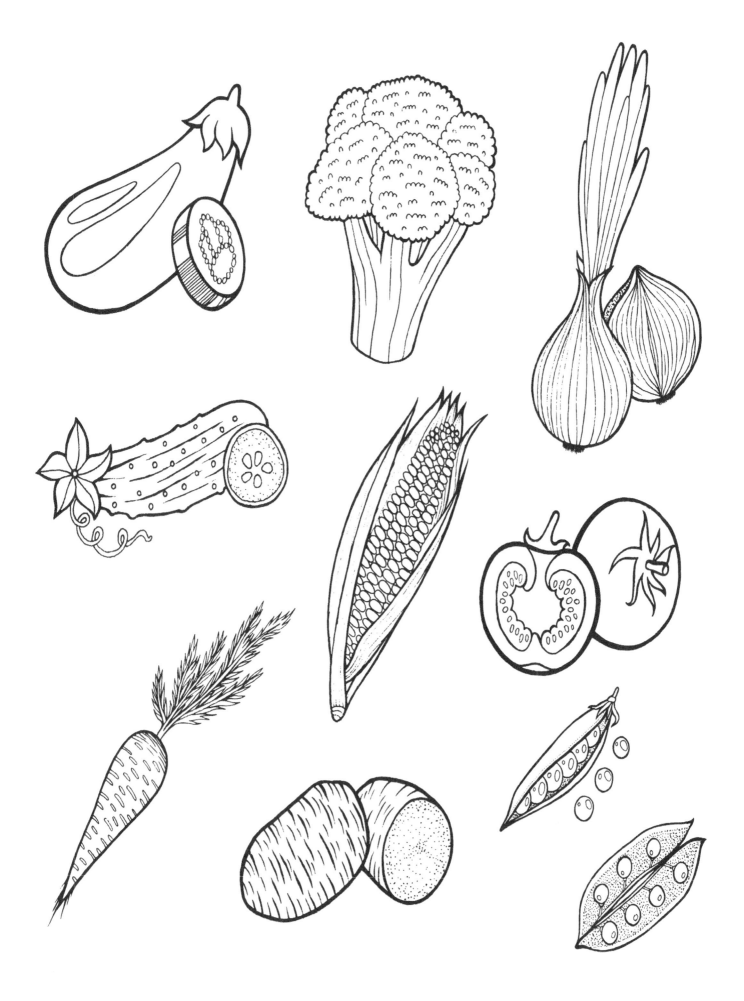

The Garden is Rich

The garden is rich with diversity
With plants of a hundred families
In the space between the trees
With all the colours and fragrances.
Basil, mint and lavender,
Great Mystery keep my remembrance pure,
Raspberry, Apple, Rose,
Great Mystery fill my heart with love,
Dill, anise, tansy,
Holy winds blow in me.
Rhododendron, zinnia,
May my prayer be beautiful
May my remembrance O Great Mystery
Be as incense to thee
In the sacred grove of eternity
As I smell and remember
The ancient forests of earth
— Chinook Psalter

How You Can Help Keep Our Traditions Alive

- November is Native American History month and celebrated throughout the United States to remember our heritage and share our rich history with story telling and events.
- To learn more about Native American History visit the museum or view online.
- National Museum of the Native American- Smithsonian https://americanindian.si.edu/
- Document Land Acknowledgement: Native Americans were the first people to live in places we call "home" in the United States. Many names of states, towns, and cities have Native American meanings. One way we can continue our Native American culture and traditions is to discover which tribes originally were located across the country. For example, the land we live on in New Jersey is from the Nanticoke Lenni Lenape tribe, so we acknowledge our land as Lenape. Researching your land acknowledgment is a great way to continue our history. You can learn more here: https://native-land.ca/
- Celebrate Indigenous People's Day: Read books by Native American writers, listen to tribal music, or share an amazing recipe. Sharing the history of indigenous peoples and their special stories keeps their memories with us.
- Include Native traditions in celebrations, such as adding these recipes to your Thanksgiving gatherings.
- Attend local cultural rituals and festivals. Around the country, over 500 tribes gather to celebrate the seasons, the harvest, and the changes of the moon. Powwows offer traditional music, clothing, dances, and food in communities for everyone to share our culture. My family attends Powwows in New Jersey and Delaware in the early summer.
- Respect the Earth: plant your own food, recycle, and trying not to be wasteful are all great ways to respect our land.
- Honor Native Americans by showing respect to our culture. Avoid jokes or images that portray our heritage in a negative way. Many times, when people think of Native Americans, they do so in ways that can be hurtful or untrue to our heritage. It is important to not wear our clothing as a costume or comment on historic facts that may be upsetting. Sharing the true history and the great contributions of our culture is a great way to keep negative stories from creating false or mean language that is harmful or untrue.
- Create your own traditions by sharing these recipes with your family and enjoy our rich history by spending time with your ancestors.

About the Author

Dr. June grew up in South Jersey, where she loved music and movies and aspired to travel and work in her favorite place, New York City. Her mom loved to sew and cook, and her father loved cars and worked at her grandfather's garage on the weekends. The garage became the location for her mommom's market. Her father would bring fresh fruit and vegetables home each weekend, where her mother would prepare recipes for the family to enjoy. Her favorite time of year was the Christmas holiday, when she would gather with her cousins and celebrate with food and traditions that are still used today.

As she followed her passion for learning, she attended Montclair State College (University), achieving a BA in Marketing while she continued to cherish her heritage by traveling and storytelling. She has an MBA in Management from Strayer University and a Doctorate of Education from Wilmington University in Organizational Leadership and Innovation where she focused her dissertation work on diversity and cultural initiatives.

She spent years in corporate positions traveling and working in New York before transitioning to a role as Executive Director for the American Red Cross before moving on to Dean of Lifelong Learning at Rowan College at Burlington County. Currently, Dr. June is the Statewide Diversity Leadership Officer for the Center for Family Services. She provides cultural competency leadership for mental health and addiction agencies throughout New Jersey, using her own experience with diversity and culture to ensure that her staff and clients are respected and valued.

Dr. June received her Native American name from the Nanticoke Lenni-Lenape tribe, located in Bridgeton, New Jersey, as part of a sacred ceremony when tribe members are presented to the Creator. Her Native American name is Charging Spirit, based on her energy, positive aura, drive, and determination. Her name was presented to her by her husband, Michael, and cousin Gail Gould. This honor will reflect her spirit throughout her life and guard her cultural journey in the clan.

She is a lifelong resident of New Jersey. She loves to spend time with her husband, Michael, and adult daughter, Alyssa, along with their furry kids, the dogs Charlie Fredward and Chanel, Bean the cat, and Bubbles the turtle.
Contact Dr. DePonte Sernak at LinkedIn at www.linkedin.com/in/dr-june-deponte-sernak or at jsernak@gmail.com.

Made in the USA
Middletown, DE
01 November 2023

41650599R00031